A CALM AND QUIET MIND

Simple advice for beginning meditators.

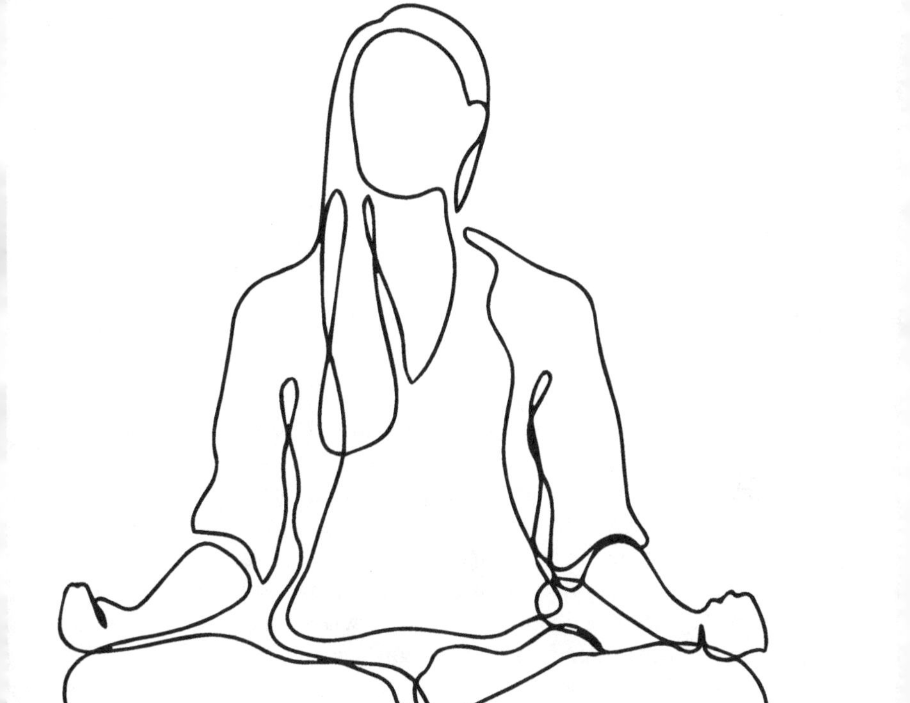

SHELBI BAILOR L.AC. MSTOM

For permission requests, write to the author at: shelbiabailor@gmail.com

A Calm And Quiet Mind / Shelbi Bailor L.Ac. MSTOM—1st ed.

Paperback: 978-1-956989-11-3
Hardcover: 978-1-956989-12-0

Introduction

I run a busy acupuncture clinic in Chicago. In my work as an acupuncturist, I've watched interest in meditation blossom over the years. More than ever, clients mention that they meditate or do mindfulness practices.

Recently, I became curious about what my clients meant when they mentioned meditation and mindfulness. I started digging a little deeper and asking more questions. These casual conversations sparked my curiosity, as the answers were so varied.

Most conversations would start with the client saying something along the lines of "I really should meditate" or "I know I should do my mindfulness practice." It was also common for them to tack on, "but my mind is too busy," before I could even ask my next questions.

My follow-up questions were, "What kind of practice do you do?" and "Where did you learn it?"

Of all the people I asked, no one had formal training. Most were using apps, following advice from someone on YouTube, or were working with something they learned in yoga. Few had a daily practice that they could describe. None had goals in meditation (some thought meditation should be without goals). None could specifically state how they would know if they had experienced growth in a meditation practice.

My idea of a meditation practice did not match up with what any of my clients described.

Of course, this small sample size of people was in no way a formal study, but it was enough to spark my interest. I kept thinking it was so strange that the words meditation and mindfulness were familiar enough to be used in regular conversation but too vague to be useful as actual practice for most of these clients.

I started to think that marketplace overwhelm may be to blame. With all of these notions about meditation out in the world, perhaps the stricter versions of these ideas, promoted initially among yogis and monastics who were devoting their lives to meditation, had been watered down and used as fodder for influencers and advertising agencies. I started to suspect that instead of helping people through meditative practices, the marketplace may be serving little more than to confuse people by offering an endless buffet of spirituality. Leaving everyone stuffed but still undernourished.

This simple book about meditation is an attempt to bridge that gap. I want meditation to nourish you. To have a practice that feels like a real meal rather than a bunch of deserts. For this to happen, you need to be clear on where you are going with your meditation, and how to set yourself up for success.

I believe the practice of meditation should be simple. Not easy. I would never claim that. But simple.

Hundreds of belief systems and lineages from around the

world, spanning thousands of years, have meditative aspects to them, from Yogic traditions coming out of the Indus valley, to Mahayana traditions in northern India and Tibet, to Zen traditions in Korea and Japan, and finally, to the Theravada traditions of Southeast Asia. Even Islam and Christianity have contemplative sects with meditative components, the Sufis and mystics.

With all the various types of meditation, it can often feel mysterious or even complicated. It may even make it hard to know where to begin. When you get down to it, the instructions for any meditation practice amount to only a page or two. The practice itself is rarely complex.

You could learn how to do just about any meditation technique in 5 minutes.

As simple as instructions on meditation are, it's what happens when you actually meditate that prompts people to write volumes.

This book is longer than two pages because the mind gets really noisy when you sit down to meditate. Sticking to even the barest-bones instructions is a tricky task, especially since mastery of even the simplest technique can take a lifetime. Even the simplest technique is hard to master without any context.

The possibilities in meditation are akin to climbing Mt. Everest. The higher you go, the less company you keep. The majority of people aren't trying to make it to the top of Everest but may at least enjoy getting further than the crowded and noisy marketplace below. With what I offer in this book, you can rise above the marketplace and get established at base camp. I consider base camp in terms of meditation traditions as access concentration. This is the first step, not to be skipped, in achieving mastery over your own mind. It seems that the majority of people don't even know that it's possible to make it that far, mostly because they have not received directions.

My Beginnings in Meditation

I started meditating over 20 years ago.

Rather than dip my toes in, I dove into meditation practice by starting with a 10-day silent retreat outside Dharamsala, India. What began as a challenge among backpackers in Turkey turned into a lifelong practice.

I learned and practiced a simple meditation technique for at least 8 hours each of the ten days I was there. And then, I went on to attend silent meditation courses whenever I had the chance.

It probably goes without saying that it was my first time being silent for longer than a day if that—no books, journals, phones, computers, and no chatting with friends or fellow meditators. We were allowed to speak with the teacher if we had questions about meditation and to speak with the manager if we had questions or concerns about health or accommodations. That was it. My only entertainment for those ten days was a family of monkeys. They would play on the tin roof of the meditation hall all afternoon, only taking a break to stare at the meditators on the way to the dining hall.

What happens in silent meditation retreats is almost impossible to replicate in daily life. In retreat, without continuous input from the rest of the world, it becomes easier to focus the mind on the object of meditation. In retreat, you are left with thoughts of the past that bubble up, projections for the future that compel you forward, but mostly, the task of being present. These hours without distraction allow for the meditation practice to become solidified and for the meditator to get over the initial hurdles of meditation and into some deeper, life-changing states.

Since my meditation practice went from absolutely zero to 10 days of silence, I thought that was the best way to go about learning to meditate. Like most who find something that works for them, I was ready to shout it from the rooftops and have every person I met to sign up to sit a 10-day course. Needless to say, my enthusiasm did not parallel the people around me. I have to admit now that my 25-year-old zest for the meditator's life may have been annoying.

Life is Complicated and Busy

As I grew my acupuncture practice in Chicago, I still felt that meditation could cure all ills. However, I was starting to see that for my clients, a 10-day trip to a silent meditation course, sitting on the floor, eating vegetarian food, and spending hours alone with their minds was not a vacation suited to most. People I work with have busy lives, professions, families, and pets. If they can carve out the time, most choose a relaxing vacation, complete with comfortable beds, great food, and cocktails. I can't blame anyone for that.

For many years, I let it go. My meditation practice was my own thing; it made me better as a practitioner. My best reviews say, "Shelbi has a calming presence." That presence is courtesy of daily meditation. I stopped thinking of it as something I should encourage clients to do.

My own life became complicated and busy too. I have had to adapt my meditation practice over the years to accommodate my daughter's life stages. My two-hour daily practice is sometimes whittled down to a lean 10 minutes, depending on her waking, sleeping, and school schedule. At a certain point, the dog, the business, and becoming a single mom myself made it almost impossible to carve out that time. Still, meditation has been a consistent companion in the 20-plus years since I started. No matter what life throws my way. I always return to my practice.

Over the past couple of years, my clients, like everyone in the world, have been challenged in ways that none of us expected. Living through a global pandemic has brought life's uncertainty to the forefront of our minds. More than ever, I am treating people for anxiety, grief, and depression. Now more than ever, I think it is worth it for all people to find strategies that help mitigate some of the worry that has rooted itself in our way of being. Creating mental resilience is needed at this time in the world.

Especially now, many would find it impossible to attend a meditation retreat, but we need meditation more than ever. I finally feel like it is worth it for me to share what I know of meditation and to encourage people to meditate, even if they aren't interested in diving into the deep end as I did.

Who Am I To Write a Book About Meditation?

I may not be qualified to write this book. To be honest, it took me a while to feel right about doing so. In the world of meditation, there are people who get permission to teach only after they have made it through various attainments or have been part of communities for a long time. I know and respect those people.

There are people who have steeped themselves in Monastic life for decades, who have far more experience than I do. They are super qualified to write books on meditation. Many of them have.

Some people have PhDs and come at it from an academic angle. I respect the work it took them to achieve that status.

I'm none of those things. I'm a person who has practiced meditation for over 20 years. I have studied with many teachers from different lineages but have been committed to one practice for the majority of that time. That long-term personal relationship to that practice, which has included study and integration of the concepts into my life, is what I've got to offer.

That, and what is absolutely true for me: I've put in some serious cushion time.

Having a twenty-plus-year relationship with this particular discipline without being a nun means that I have had to work with meditation as part of daily life in this very modern world.

I know what it's like to have a messy life full of noise and complications. I don't carry out my daily practice in some idyllic setting anymore. I live on the third floor of a brownstone in Chicago, situated at the crossroads of a highly trafficked street and alley. All day long, there are garbage trucks and delivery trucks navigating the tight alley. Not only are they noisy, but they sometimes make the building shake. In summer, small groups hang out on the corner below, partying and listening to music. The city sounds of sirens are a regular occurrence.

I'm not complaining. I live in the city. If quiet were a requirement, I would never meditate.

I also share time with a dog. Not an easygoing one. I share time with a dog who should live in the country, roaming free, herding sheep. He objects to me meditating or doing anything that doesn't give him my undivided attention. Sometimes he wants to be on the cushion with me (I call that dogitation).

In addition to this pet who objects strongly to my meditation practice, I have a kid, a business where I see about 40 clients a week, and a boyfriend, none of whom care if I become enlightened as long as they are fed, loved, and given my support in life and healing.

This is another reason I feel compelled to write this book. Coming from the far extreme of devoting big portions of my life to meditation to incorporating it into a life that is often more about helping others gives me this perspective. I understand where you may be coming from if a committed meditation practice feels out of reach. I do get it.

I may not be qualified to teach you the very highest levels of meditation from the vantage point of a forest monastery, but I can help bridge the confusing gap between the noisy meditation marketplace, helping you get beyond the initial hurdles that all meditators face. I hope to help you see that you can start practicing wherever you are and under your circumstances.

A teacher once said to me that you only need to know more than your student in order to teach. This is a book for beginners. I have spent hours and hours wrangling my own mind into concentration, and I feel that I can offer you some help in doing the same.

How to Use this Book

After interviewing clients, it became clear that the best way to help people get started on a home practice would be by writing simple and clear advice without fluff. With a book like this, it feels tempting to spend words proving myself or giving some sort of reference to other works. In fact, at one point, this book was a 50,000-word document.

After interviewing a client, a busy single mom with three kids, I joked and said I should write a children's book for adults. She applauded the idea and said, "Shelbi, I love you and want to meditate, but there is no way I am finding the extra time to read 50,000 words. Give me 500, and I may be able to find the time to meditate." At the end of the day, I want you to spend more time with your butt on the cushion than with your nose in the book.

Obviously, this book is longer than 500 words, but I did take this heavily into consideration, working on cutting it down to the simplest and clearest format possible.

After this introduction, I will be as succinct, with as few words per page as possible so that you can take in this information and use it with little confusion. If it reads like I'm being bossy, it's because I am trying to save words. (Also, I am kind of a bossy person, just ask my dog.)

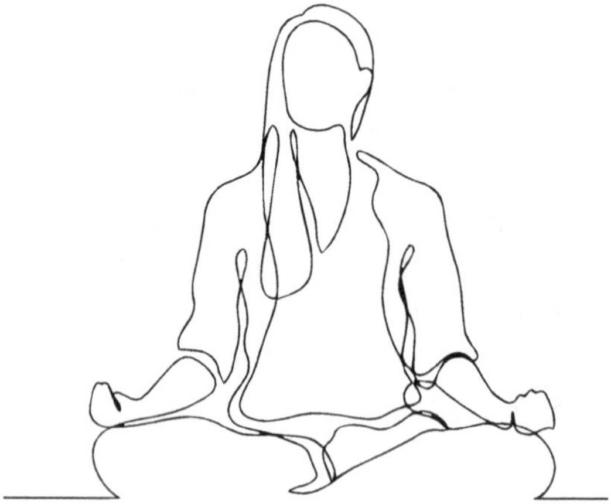

This Book is Broken Down into Three Parts:

THE WHAT AND WHY, THE PRACTICE, AND ADVANCED CONSIDERATIONS

If you are tired of looking at words, just go to part 2 and get started. The benefits of meditation come only from practicing. Any other knowledge is gravy. You learn meditation by doing it.

PART 1
THE WHAT AND WHY

Learn what makes something meditation and what does not, why you should do it, and some basics and background to get started.

PART 2
THE PRACTICE

Set up a home practice with simple instructions.

PART 3
GOING DEEPER AND UNDERSTANDING THE CONTEXT.

Understand what comes next as your practice gets stronger. Navigate life through the lens of meditation practice.

My Hope

With consistent, diligent, and sincere effort, you can create a home meditation practice that gets you beyond the initial hurdles that beginning meditators face. My wish with this book is to give you what you need to start a home practice.

You may want to take it further and get formal instructions from a living teacher or a center down the line. However, if all of that seems like too much right now, you can still grow in your meditation by sitting regularly and with the intention of growing in your ability to quiet your mind.

My wish for you is that these practices help you build mental resilience as you face your own life, that by learning how to work with your own mind and thoughts, you grow in your own peace and compassion, and that naturally, that compassion extends to those around you and out into the world.

PART 1

THE WHAT AND WHY

Defining Meditation

The world is full of spiritual, psychological, and healing approaches. Sometimes these are mistaken for meditation. Some could be considered meditation. For the purposes of this book, we're going to operate from this specific definition.

Meditation is a discipline in which you train your mind to rest quietly on the chosen object of concentration and to, within the timeframe of the session, remain neutral about any experiences that arise in the mind and body that may disrupt quiet focus.

Meditation is the Practice not the Outcome

Many people think of words like enlightenment, peace, non-attachment, or calm when they think of meditation.

While all those ideas relate to meditation and surround the culture of meditation, they are more descriptive of the outcomes than the actual practice.

Something that works really well in meditation (and in life) is to stay focused on the work rather than the outcome.

As your skills in meditation increase, you will find out how it impacts your life.

Important lessons and side effects naturally arise if you sit down and practice.

Meditation is Solitary Even When You are Surrounded by People

You have a mind, and you have a consistent object of meditation. The breath.

These you carry with you everywhere.

No one else can fully know your mind. No one else can feel your every breath.

You are in charge of healing your life through the discipline of training your own mind.

You will have friends and helpers along the way. You will experience love and closeness with partners, family members, or pets in your life.

That said, no one else can be in charge of your mind and the decisions you make with it.

You are the leader of this kingdom, in charge of how you use the resources of your mind, body, and breath.

Your time on the planet is only yours to use.

Meditation practice is your time to change your own mind.

Meditation is a Discipline and not Always Easy

Sitting Ain't for Sissies.

Meditation is a deliberate practice that you take on in order to meet the world without the filter of your normally reactive mind.

Rather than seeking to feel good or running from feeling bad, you train your mind in the discipline of being with life exactly as it is.

Sometimes life is comfortable and wonderful.

Sometimes life is hard and painful.

Meditation teaches us to face life as it is. Facing what is painful is a bold act.

Learning to avoid the enticement of temporary pleasures. Equally bad ass.

This takes courage. You are capable.

Meditation Takes Concentration

We train to focus the mind on a certain object to the exclusion of everything else.

In some traditions that object is outside the body. Like on the flame of a candle, a prayer or mantra, or a passage from a scripture.

Here, we will learn concentration as a part of a larger practice.

There are three parts of this practice;

Lifestyle. Concentration. Wisdom. Traditionally known as

Sila, Samadhi, and Panna.

All three trainings simultaneously support and depend on each-other. But none of them happen without the ability to stabilize the mind.

Concentration is basecamp.

Meditation Trains Us to Notice What Our Minds are Doing

We adopt a special way of seeing in meditation.

We learn to see a thought as a thought.

Meditation guides us to overcome the habit of believing the content of our thoughts as some separate and important entity.

This dismantles their power to make us feel some type of way.

Normally, in waking life, we tend to attach to thoughts as though they are truth.

Our thoughts tell stories that we become invested in, thinking that they represent who we are and what the world is.

These thoughts and perceptions are generated through filters.

As we interact with waking reality through our senses,quickly, before we know it, our minds start to generate a storied interpretation of what is happening.

This is almost always based on habits from past conditioning.

Thoughts tell us that the interpretation is the reality.

Meditation trains us to resist the temptation to believe those thoughts.

Meditation at its Core is not Religious

You don't need to be Buddhist, Hindu, or Taoist to meditate.

You can also relax any fears you have that meditation goes against your religious beliefs.

Here, we work with meditation only as a system of training your mind.

Many of these meditation traditions intersect with religious beliefs and culture of the places where they are practiced. You will see people doing rituals and offerings with opening prayers and chants.

Some practices still carry the aesthetics of earlier times, such as the Tibetan traditions incorporating shamanic or animist elements, or the Japanese traditions carrying forth some aspects of Shinto.

That said, cultural appropriation is not necessary for meditation.

Respect for lineage is encouraged. You can only get so far without understanding the historical and cultural context of any practice you take on, but even when you know more, the actual work stays the same.

You do not need to adopt a new religion to train your mind.

Meditation is an Awesome and Worthy Endeavor

Your mind directs your life. Who knows where an undisciplined mind will take you? Seems like a good idea to take charge of that. Am I right?

MEDITATION IS NOT...

Crystals and Gong Baths and Reiki Oh My!

The modern world offers up a heavily marketed spiritual buffet. With all of this sparkling press it's easy to mistake anything related to energy work or healing with meditation.

There are all sorts of wonderful practices we seek out in this era that are derived from ancient traditions. They help us to enjoy states of relaxation and bliss. They facilitate spiritual opening and connection.

From shamanic journeys, to Reiki, to chakra healings, the world is ripe with options for spiritual growth.

Many of these help us heal, they expand our intuition, give us visions, and help us see the mythic nature of ourselves.

There are healing practices that others do for us, guided visualizations, acupuncture, shiatsu, craniosacral, energy work, massage, crystal healing.

These amazing practices are encouraged as self care and healing. Sometimes they result in meditative states.

Still though, they are not meditation.

Meditative results facilitated by outside influences are not the same as having a sustainable meditation practice that you facilitate for yourself.

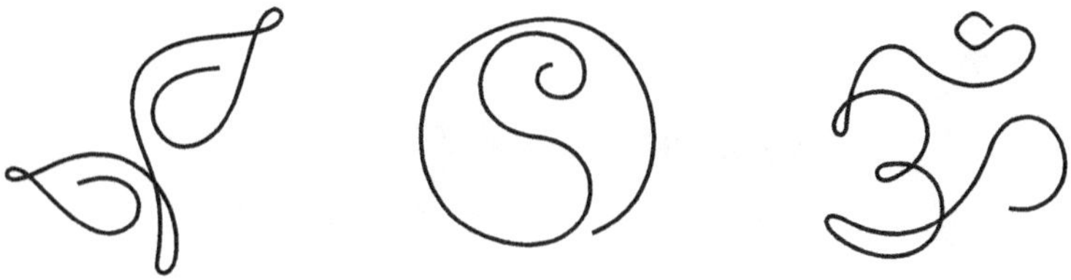

A Time to Remember

Thinking about the past, getting lost in stories, rehashing traumas and conversations, going over them again and again.

Sometimes cushion time seems like a great opportunity to think about all that has happened before.

Rumination is one of the mind's favorite hobbies.

Given any quiet time, those memories go really wild! Storytime on steroids!

While it may seem great to finally get the chance to fix the unfixable, that's not what you are sitting down to do.

Getting caught up in the content is a task better left to other times.

Therapy, journaling, or talking with friends, are great ways to work with the stories that are in the mind. Anything important that comes up will still be there after your session. You can believe that! Feel free to write it all down for analysis after your meditation session.

Future, Trippin, and Fantasizing

Done fixing the past? Moving on to planning the future?

The mind will have you believe that the best use of your meditation session is to dream up a future that delivers you from all your problems.

In this future you are the dazzling hero of those stories. Grandiosity galore!

You may have heard about meditation as a way to manifest things.

While it is true that a strong and clear mind can help you build a better life for yourself, that is not the purpose of sitting practice.

That life isn't out "there" somewhere. It's built on a foundation of clarity and calm intent right here and now.

Don't put the cart before the horse.

Sit down and meditate to get that strong clear mind. Dream about your future later.

While not meditating you can make lists, manifestation maps, journal out the perfect day, week, and month. Hire a life or career coach. Light a candle for your future, do a ceremony, or pray. Use that calm mind for good.

A Soft and Fuzzy Warm Experience. A Fluffy New Age-y Blanket

You may be attracted to meditation because you want to soften life's hard edges, or in some way be delivered from suffering. It is true that meditation will often offer this to you. There are some pretty cool states of bliss that happen for serious meditators. But the practice of meditation is razor sharp.

You are not getting into the practice to make your mind fuzzy and diffuse.

You are a spiritual warrior on the cushion sharpening your weapon of mental specificity.

You are honing skills, becoming a master of your own mind.

Try not to confuse the potential results with the actual practice.

Some Vague Practice

Meditation is not some generally amorphous practice that came from somewhere in the east.

Hmm. Was it India? Burma? China?

Any meditation practice started somewhere, likely a long time ago. Most practices were designed for monks and delivered highly specific training with detailed maps of what would happen in the mind of the meditator on the way to enlightenment.

Those practices and instructions are still relevant and important for us today even if we have new obstacles to contend with. We still are working with the same basic equipment. A human body and mind.

Whatever practice you choose, focus on the actual practice while on the cushion, but enjoy researching and finding out more about the tradition or lineage that your practice comes from during other times of the day.

A Way to Let Yourself off the Hook

One of the modern western layers we have put on meditation is that we should go easy on ourselves.

Perhaps this has come as a reaction to our cultural tendency to be "control enthusiasts," as one teacher calls it. We want to use meditation to balance out any conservative tendencies that have been overly influential in our lives. Meditation seems "groovy" compared to some of our strict religious upbringings.

Meditation is not an opportunity to coddle your emotions.

In sincere practice, we are always calibrating to the place, which offers enough tension without pushing it too far.

While judgment and self-flagellation don't help a true practice, discipline and accountability do.

Balance puts practice in its natural order. Find that perfect point between pushing yourself and being kind toward your limitations.

Once you get past a certain point in your practice, there will be times when you enjoy the ease of just being without any thought. But that ease does not come from taking it easy.

Just like we don't give a trophy to both the winning and the losing team, there is a reason we put in the work to achieve something.

If it were too easy, it wouldn't be rewarding.

Flat Abs and Perky Buns

In fact, sitting for hours on end may result in flat buns and not-so-perky abs.

It is easy to think that someone who is advanced in meditation will look or behave like some sort of Adonis-type figure with a steady gaze and perfected persona.

Not usually. Meditators come in all shapes, sizes, and ages. Meditators come from different socio-economic backgrounds and cultures around the world.

No need to get wrapped up in having the identity of a meditator, adopting an external appearance that makes you look enlightened.

You can meditate and work toward mastery and freedom over your life, wearing whatever you choose.

While on the cushion that will likely resemble pajamas.

Maybe they will be organic cotton; maybe they will have Marvel Characters on them.

You do you.

If there is any quality that most advanced meditators have, it's calm alertness. If you want that vibe, go get it, tiger! Get on that cushion!

WHY MEDITATE?

So far, this sounds like a whole lot of work. Discipline, commitment, not getting to wear a cute enlightenment outfit... I'm really not selling this am I? Why in the world would anybody bother taking the time to do this.

The Clinical Reasons to Meditate

A quick google search will let you know that there are all sorts of amazing health benefits from meditation.

The Mayo Clinic Cites the following;

Gaining a new perspective on stressful situations.
Building skills to manage your stress.
Increasing self awareness.
Reducing negative emotions.
Increasing imagination and creativity.
Increasing patience and tolerance.

These very clinical sounding cliff-notes should be enough to convince you, however, there are some even cooler reasons to meditate, some have been proven by science, and some anecdotal.

BRAIN WAVES: SCIENCE BACKED REASONS TO MEDITATE

Amygdala Shrinkage

It may seem counterintuitive to celebrate any region of the brain shrinking; however, having a less prominent amygdala results in living a more peaceful life.

The amygdala is part of the brain, sometimes referred to as the lizard brain.

It contributes to emotional processing and is the first step on the road to recognizing and responding to danger.

It is responsible for fear, stress, and anger.

The amygdala is always scanning the horizon for threats, whether true or perceived. Once noticing a threat, the amygdala sends a distress signal to the hypothalamus, setting off a cascade of signals that prepare our body to either fight or flee the situation.

In multiple studies, meditators and non-meditators had disturbing images shown to them. The amygdalas of meditators responded slowly, allowing them to recognize the image as an image before setting up that cascade of stress responses that would tell the body to respond to a real threat.

Normally our amygdala sets the reaction in motion before we have even had time to process what we see. This remarkable benefit of meditation is especially important in the modern world when we often respond to images and emotions, not life or death situations.

Having less lizard brain allows us to be more human and compassionate as we grow in our ability to listen and enjoy others around us without being constantly triggered.

Less amygdala means coming out of a chronically stressed and hyperstimulated state.

Imagine the benefits of operating as more human and less lizard!

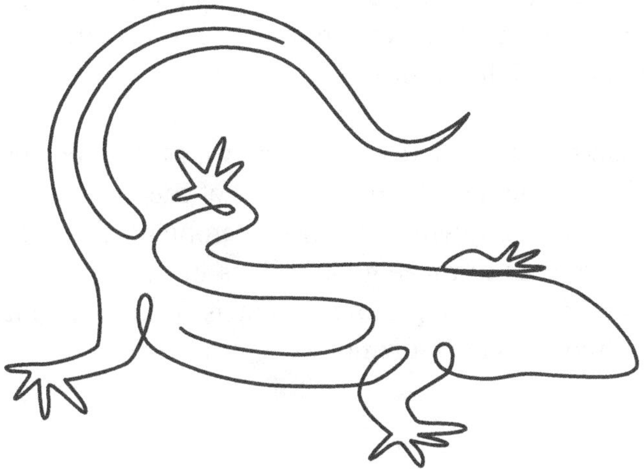

Gamma Growth

Gamma waves have the fastest frequency of all brain waves and are the key to enlightened states of mind and inner peace.

Experienced meditators are more likely than most to experience these impressive brain waves.

Neuroscientists have hooked up serious meditations to scalp electrodes to study what happens. Meditation masters have a higher prevalence of gamma in their minds and are more likely to access gamma states in everyday life outside of cushion time.

Studies into the effects of meditation on our brains indicate that when our brain is functioning in Gamma frequencies, it is able to create new pathways in the brain for neurons to flow in between. This indicates that our information is being communicated differently than normal.

This Gamma wave increase is where we get to enjoy pushing into the frontiers of the possibilities of the human brain. At this powerful frequency, the brain can heighten perception, empowering us to make great strides in our inner development and experience profound compassion. They contribute to inspired problem-solving.

What About Alpha?

Alpha brain waves are the prominent waves for states of wakeful rest.

These waves are activated in moments throughout the day when you are not engaged in problem-solving or performing mentally taxing tasks, when you have completed your chores and work for the day, or in the moments when you first wake up before you start thinking about all you need to do.

Alpha waves are present when we reach this sort of state of relaxation. We are still alert and able to function, but we do not feel stress or pressure related to what we are doing.

These states contribute to rest and relaxation. Alpha wave dominance can be achieved through other activities and is a bit of lower hanging fruit than achieving dominant gamma states. However, meditation is one way to activate the alpha wave and contribute to less anxiety and stress response in the brain.

Allowing Life

A regular meditation practice will help you see how often you exert influence over situations that are better left alone.

Brains like to worry, problem-solve, and attempt control.

When you sit down to meditate, you see the thoughts for what they are. You learn from direct experience that they are largely inconsequential.

With that understanding, you get better at taking a pause before interrupting the flow of life.

Those issues you think you should worry about are so often not even the problems you really need to solve.

Meditation teaches us to be with what is actually happening so we can keep our eye on the ball.

The problems of life are moving targets. Without training, the mind will treat thoughts as problems, putting out attention in the wrong place.

Meditation teaches us to keep our attention in the moment where it is most useful.

Allow for better possibilities.

Subtle Happiness

By training your mind toward living in the present moment, you have more opportunities everyday to be awake to the world around you. Consistent and diligent meditation practice allows you to see the world as more than just an opportunity to get what you want or avoid what you don't.

This offers up "subtle happiness" a state of contentment that is available even when circumstances are less than your version of ideal.

When your mind is clear and open, your senses have an increased ability to enjoy the nuanced beauty of the natural world. Colors are more vibrant, sounds and smells more potent. You can enjoy the day just as it is.

When we are swept up in our mental and emotional dramas, our senses are blocked.

Somewhat tender, subtle happiness is a state that needs protection from the storms of emotion, like a little sapling that needs protection as it grows. Meditation is the fence that protects that state of mind.

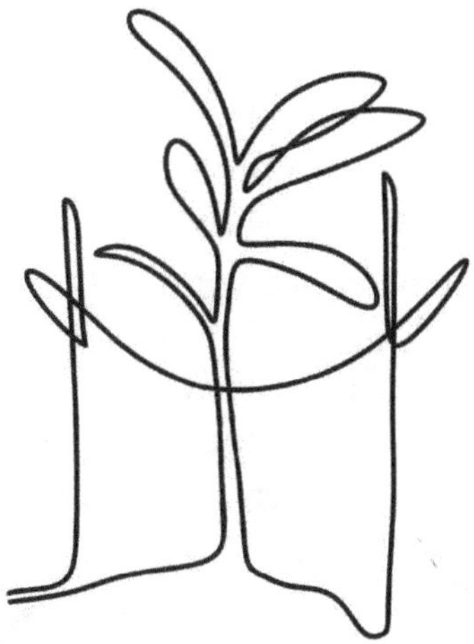

Skillful Days

When you adhere to a consistent and deliberate meditation practice, you automatically become your own teacher.

That commitment will show you what works in life and what doesn't.

Showing up to the cushion with a gossip hangover will teach you to avoid negativity.

Showing up to the cushion with an alcohol hangover will teach you to avoid substances.

Those moments when you sit down to train your mind, you also, invariably, get a glimpse of what is going on in your life. Stuff will come up, and you tend to it while on the cushion by watching it and then returning to the object of meditation.

Here it may seem like a contradiction since you know better than to get swept up in the content of your problems. Those problems that come up for you are not meant to be solved intellectually while you are there, but they will arise anyway.

As they do, you will train yourself away from making more trouble for yourself by your behavior. Consistent practice leads to a better life, and a less chaotic life leads to strength in meditation.

True Freedom Of Direction

A friend and long-time meditator cited freedom as his number one reason for meditating.

Our cultural conditioning and bias are so deeply embedded in our subconscious that most of the time, even when we think we are making choices in life, those choices are coming from conditioning rather than the present moment.

As you grow in meditation, you learn to see the moving and changing nature of your thoughts. With enough practice, you will even start to see how an experience hits your senses, gets a reaction from you and how the thoughts are excess layers of noise on top of that conditioned reaction.

At a certain point, having established the vantage point of being a non-reactive watcher, you become less likely to respond like a puppet to your social and cultural conditioning. You literally "free your mind."

You respond as your true self.

On a conscious level, you may believe you are in charge of your life and making decisions as an autonomous adult. If you don't have mastery over your mind, you don't have mastery over your life.

Being in Step with TIme

In Classical Chinese Medicine, we understand that there is constant movement in our systems. Our physical bodies stay healthy and alive all day and every day by responding to the environment around us: the rhythms of day and night, the change of the seasons, and the need for food, water, and sleep. We are always in a push and pull, getting our needs met with the resources available.

Good health dictates itself by being "right with time." That means we are in sync with natural rhythms and can change and adapt in real-time to stay healthy.

When bogged down by too much of anything or when depleted from being over-extended, our bodies stop keeping up with the timing of life, leading to illness or discomfort.

Our mental and emotional states are part of this balancing act.

A daily meditation practice allows us to process what is happening but not just on our usual conscious level. Like emotional housekeeping, by becoming less attached to the content of the thoughts, we filter out the unnecessary. We do not get bogged down with a stockpile of unprocessed emotion. We stop spending energy on things that don't serve us.

IS IT THE RIGHT TIME TO TAKE ON A MEDITATION PRACTICE?

Maybe Not

Now that you see what a meditation practice looks like, you may wonder if trying to build a consistent practice is right for you at this time in your life.

Honestly, it may not be.

There are obvious reasons that people think they can't take on a home practice. Not having time is the most common.

It is hard to find the time. Similar to deciding when to fit exercise into your day, carving out a window of opportunity to stick with a sitting practice takes maneuvering. There will be plenty of days where it feels more important to do the dishes, call your long-lost auntie or bathe your chinchilla.

One way to get over this is to be open to times you might not have considered. Obviously, the morning is best. If you can wake up early and get it done right away, you are less likely to get caught up in other obligations.

For parents, it may make more sense to meditate after dropping kids off and before work, if that is possible, or around lunch or early afternoon.

Every time of day has its own challenges. Stay flexible, stay committed; it's worth it to give yourself the chance.

In the end, time may be the easiest obstacle to overcome.

Don't Meditate

One serious meditation friend said, "tell them not to meditate." He thought I should name my book Don't Meditate.

Ok, maybe it seems a bit snobby to say something like that, but his reasoning came from a compassionate place.

He is someone who has meditated enough to qualify for brain studies (he had those electrodes attached to his head and went through MRIs). He knows what serious practice looks like.

He thinks that without hours of stillness and support offered by being on retreat, it may not be possible to get into the concentration states that make the whole thing worthwhile. Without that depth, in his opinion, you would lose motivation and not get anywhere that you may as well not even try.

Upon hearing this story, a few clients got a bit defiant. They wanted to prove him wrong. It was almost as if he unintentionally threw down the gauntlet. Nothing like telling people they can't do something to make them want to do it more!

To a degree, his opinion makes sense. It is hard to achieve

deep concentration when the noisy waves of daily life keep crashing down on you.

Where he is wrong–he hasn't met you!

With the right kind of effort, and by staying focused on the simple instructions, you can build your skills and get into the early stages of concentration. Even if that's as far as you ever go, you will still do better in life than if you had never tried. One of the biggest obstacles is that people don't know how to create a meditation practice designed for growth because the advertised perception of meditation is a relaxation practice.

That said, there are times when it will feel like an uphill battle to do this sort of practice. When getting a massage, phoning a friend, or calling a mental health specialist is the best action to take.

More than Normal Overwhelm

At some point, for every person, it becomes clear that life isn't all glitter and rainbow unicorn poop. Without exception, we will deal with pain and loss.

Many are drawn to meditation when times get hard.

Depending on the degree of your current suffering, the type of practice offered here may be too much.

Meditation has been marketed consistently as a way to become less anxious or as a method of overcoming suffering. At its core, that is exactly what meditation offers at a deep fundamental level.

However, those benefits don't always come right away. It isn't the best for quick and easy fixes when this or that has just lambasted your life, and you just need to feel better.

An established practice will help you weather almost any storm, but a brand new practice will be extra challenging if you are in the early stages of grief, suffering from extreme anxiety, panic disorders, or other mental health issues. When you sit down to meditate, your emotions may overwhelm you; they will magnify your thoughts.

Rather than force yourself to start now, it may help to consider some other self-care methods and circle back to this at another point in your healing. Find outside support to re-calibrate your nervous system. This may be a better time for therapy, massages, acupuncture, time in nature, or chocolate.

In the Middle of a Kundalini Awakening

We are living through extraordinary times. At this moment in history, more people than ever have the access and ability to learn practices that facilitate spiritual awakening.

Some people experience spontaneous spiritual awakening or

stumble into higher states of consciousness without having a practice or guidelines for what is happening.

There are reasons for this; often due to early childhood trauma, people have adapted mental coping strategies to "leave" the body as a way of survival. For some, it is simply that they are doing yogic or other spiritual practices that turbocharge these awakened states.

Unfortunately, some teachers can be misleading. Some have ended up in mental institutions for behavior that mimics a psychotic break.

We are rarely told in our culture to back off when we are working to achieve something. But if you are having strange experiences or feeling like the energy surging through your body is more than you can handle, it's time to pump the brakes.

In these situations, your ego may fool you into thinking that you are on the brink of enlightenment when you are becoming addicted to early meditation states that feel really "high" but are not sustainable.

If this is happening to you, stop meditating for a while. Focus on earthbound activities, exercise, massage, hugs, or cuddling pets. Eat some root vegetables or heavier, denser foods.

Seek additional support and living teachers that can help guide you.

You can resume practice at a more natural and easy pace when you are grounded.

Is it a Busy Mind or a Chaotic Life?

Ever heard or said this? "But my mind is way too busy to meditate. I've tried. I just can't do it."

Guess what? All minds are busy unless trained not to be—some more than others.

Ask yourself. Is it that your mind is too busy or that your lifestyle is too chaotic? Are you addicted to being busy?

If taking on a home practice seems impossible, first try reducing these influences in your life.

No need to overhaul everything. Just think of this as if weeding a garden. Pluck out a few problem areas and see what can blossom.

Try reducing these influences in your life.

Social Media-basically a training ground for monkey mind. Boot camp for people who want to train in perpetual distraction.

Physical Belongings- Outside clutter = inside clutter. Get your "stuff" in order. Hint, it's easier to get rid of most of it, but that's a topic for another book. As one yogi said, "I can't meditate until the carpet is vacuumed."

Alcohol-even the mildest hangover feels like concentrating through a fog. In some ways, a meditation practice can inspire you to stop drinking just by the cause-and-effect slap-on-the-wrist reality of it. At some point, you will need to choose which lifestyle is more important to you.

Relationships that inspire anger or frustration-you will have a hard time getting quiet on the cushion when stewing in perpetual irritation.

In a perfect world, you can evaluate the quality of a relationship by how equal it is in terms of your energy expenditure. Do you get back what you give? Does it lead you astray from living a peaceful life?

It may seem rude or unkind to disengage from people who take more than they give. Something we learn through a meditation practice is that we are responsible for our own choices. Again and again, we come to the cushion and work with what is present in our own minds. As you take accountability for how you contribute to discord, you recognize when others are not taking responsibility for their part in perpetuating drama.

Having a meditation practice is a sane thing to do. It is very grown up. If you know that you have some loose ends in the grown-up department, this is a great time to work on those. Learn how to communicate, and get a mediator or counselor if this is a relationship that can't be abandoned but also needs to change.

Tending to any or all of these things will set you up for a life that allows for a successful meditation practice.

For now, if you need to, set a six-month commitment to getting your life together. Circle back to creating a home practice when you have more space for it. That said, you don't need to be perfect to start meditating, not by a long shot.

Notes Before We Begin Practice

While the possibilities for growth in meditation are vast, what you experience with a simple home practice may be just the sense that you are starting to get the hang of it, that when you sit down, your mind can get into states of stillness, and that the worries that were once a cacophony are now a mild hum.

The intent for each session is that you have a few moments of suspended thinking. Where you experience a fusion of mind with your object of concentration and nothing else, even a few moments will change your mind for the better.

Base camp, for meditators, has long been known as access concentration. This is the first goal of our practice here.

There is a notion out in the world that meditation should be without goals. Closer to the truth is that placing too much emphasis on a goal that is anywhere other than the object of concentration hinders meditation. is hindered

Similar to what would happen if you were climbing a rocky mountain path complicated with tree roots and branches. If you focused only on the top of the mountain, you would trip and fall before getting very far.

You can know your destination while staying absorbed completely where you are. Think of it as an intention rather than a goal.

Fix That

A mother of six kids, a woman who garnered respect from her family, had a strategy for managing her motley crew of kids.

As soon as a snotty look or disrespectful comment was about to cross any of their faces or leave any of their mouths, she would simply look at the kid and say, "fix that."

There was no irritation, hatred, or judgment, just a simple redirection.

This is the right attitude to have toward yourself in meditation. With a basic assumption that you are worthy of your own respect and that you can win over your innate tendency to wander off, you simply fix it and move on.

Keeping the right attitude toward yourself will take you far.

Let's start meditating!

PART 2

THE HOW

Sit Down

Set Timer

Find Breath

Observe Breath

Lose Breath

Find Breath Again

Finish

Sit Down

For formal meditation practice, we sit.

While there are other options for meditation, such as walking or laying down, we don't start there.

Laying down too often ends up as nap-itating.

Walking requires a different kind of focus, the kind needed to keep us from bumping into things.

Sitting is stable and still, the posture that makes it easiest to achieve our first goal of access concentration, the state in which we can remain focused on our object of meditation with relative ease to the exclusion of other distractions for a minute or more.

Concentration will stretch into longer time periods as your meditation practice gets stronger. Until then, a minute or so is enough time to understand what it feels like to have a calm mind that allows for a gentle but resolute focus on your breath.

This may be the first stop on our path toward enlightenment, but it's also the most crucial, and skipping over it isn't an option.

Sit Indoors

Sometimes we get a fanciful notion that we should be meditating in some sort of beautiful natural setting, as is often seen in magazines. You may have noticed a common one, the silhouette of a yogi in shadow meditating while looking out over a canyon bathed in the pinks and oranges of a beautiful sunset.

As gorgeous as that is while learning to concentrate on something as subtle as the breath, sitting indoors is preferred.

Being outside offers the wind and the air and the birds and the bees... or mosquitos, too many opportunities to create a distracting sensation on your skin. You don't want to fight off predators, even tiny ones while trying to concentrate.

It will be easier to start in a temperature-controlled and wind-neutral setting. Inside.

Sit with A Straight Spine

To achieve a straight spine, stack one vertebra on top of another. Establish a vertical axis from the top of your head to the base of your spine.

With this idea in mind, use your sit bones to find stability on the bottom so that you can feel as effortless as possible in your own version of uprightness.

The truth is that none of us have a straight spine. Find that point where you sense that your skeleton supports your body, so the muscles don't hold tension to compensate.

You may have scoliosis, or you've had back surgery or something else that makes it difficult to have the same version of straight offered in anatomy textbooks. That's not a problem. You can still meditate. You've probably already found your own version of what it means to be comfortably upright. Go with that. A spine is a gift to be appreciated no matter how it deviates.

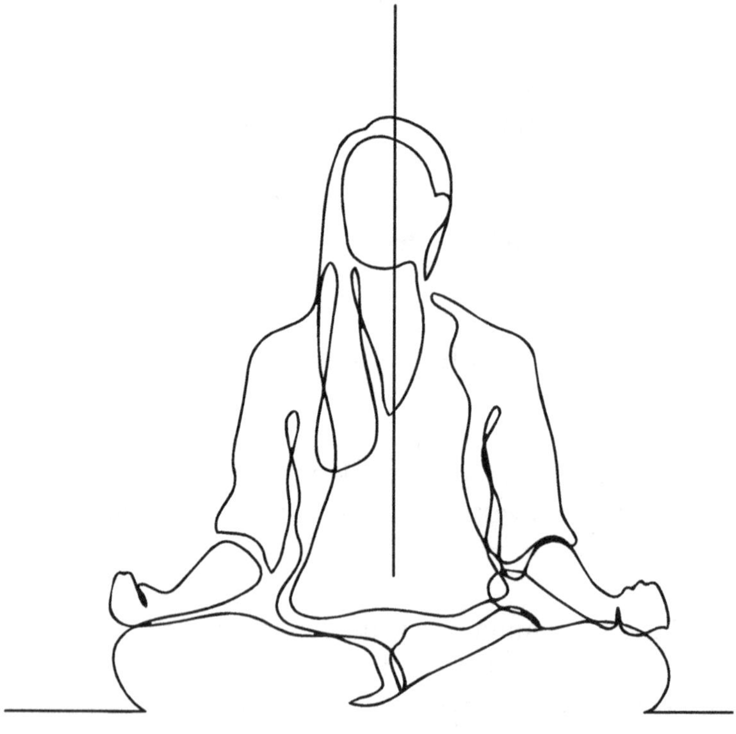

Sitting Straight Helps You Concentrate

As long as you are able to have a straight spine with the head balanced above and the sacrum comfortable below, you will have more success in holding onto a neutral and clear mental state.

There is dignity in being upright. As previously mentioned, understanding that you are worthy of self-respect is key as you learn to wrangle your mind. Sitting straight reinforces this attitude.

Find a posture that allows you to sit still for the duration of the practice.

A FEW WAYS TO SIT.

Crossed Legs

You may already have an image in your head of a meditator sitting in a cross-legged position with feet tucked in and resting on the legs. You can modify this position with the legs crossed and the feet tucked under or one foot up and one foot under.

Crossed legged position is a wonderful posture for meditation because it automatically puts the spine in a good position to be upright with a stable base.

Often this position is easier to achieve if the cushion allows the hips to be slightly higher than the knees.

For some, additional support with cushions under the knees will help.

For you, this position may not work. That's ok. There are alternate options.

Sitting While Kneeling

Kneeling is a common posture in some meditation traditions, most commonly Zen traditions coming out of Japan.

You can fold legs beneath you with your bum supported by either a meditation bench or a firm cushion.

Use a folded blanket, or a wide-based cushion called a zabuton to keep your legs from being bothered by a cold or hard floor.

Straighten the spine and keep the head lifted up off the shoulders.

Sitting on a Chair or with Props

For some, it won't work to sit cross-legged or kneel.

Pain while sitting happens for almost anyone on a longer meditation retreat sitting for hours over several days. However, some have health conditions that make sitting on the floor too painful or awkward to allow for any semblance of concentration under any circumstance.

Chair meditation is always an option and will do nothing to slow down progress as long as the spine is straight enough to allow for dignified concentration.

Watching the Waves as a Rest Posture for Prolonged Sessions

Once you have found the right position for your body, it should be no problem for you to sit for the duration of a home session that is 20 minutes or less without moving.

If you decide to take it further and sit for longer periods, subtly moving into a rest posture can help keep the meditation session going rather than succumbing to the frustration of pain.

In longer sessions, you can slowly and deliberately move into a position hugging your knees. As if sitting on the beach and watching the waves. This is a nice break and alternative if you are not ready to end the meditation session but are too uncomfortable to concentrate.

After a few moments, resume the posture that you began with.

In certain meditation traditions and for some specific practices, there are reasons to maintain posture even when the going gets rough. This is more advanced than what is offered here, but don't be surprised to encounter that discipline level should you keep growing in your meditation practice.

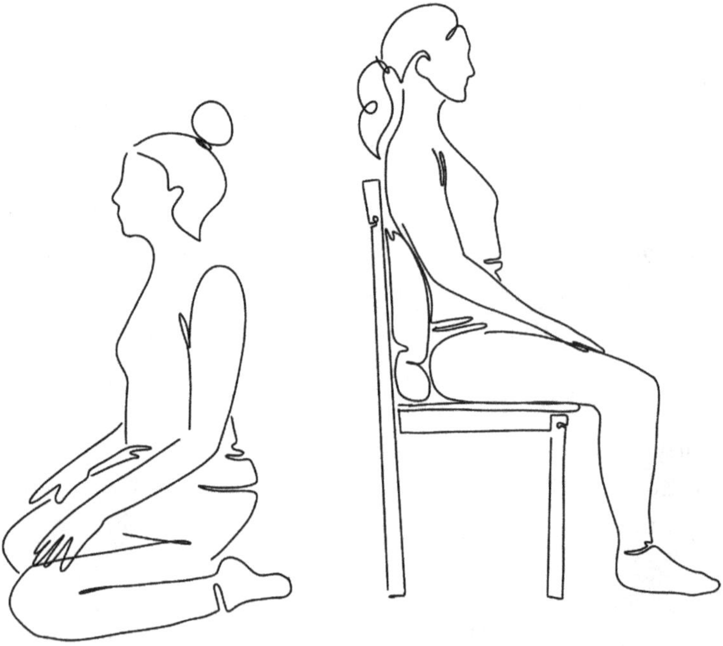

Set A Timer

Some people don't need a timer. They know when to stop naturally. These people are also in a constant state of meditation, highly trained CIA sniper agents, or something super special. They aren't mere mortals like we are.

For our practice, we need a timer.

Without a timer, there is no accountability. It is too tempting to stop meditating just because you feel like it.

The timer allows for structure around the time you meditate. It also allows time to become a non-issue. Just keep meditation going until the timer goes off.

There, now you don't need to worry about it.

HOW LONG?

In a perfect world, you would do a kick-ass two-hour-a-day practice and reach enlightenment by next year. I imagine that's asking a bit much out the gate for your home practice.

At least 20 minutes would be great, but you can start with as little as five.

You can learn techniques quickly. The instructions will be so simple. But mastering the practice will take some time, no matter how quickly you intellectually grasp the concept.

If you do too little, you won't reap the benefits.

In order to figure out a reasonable beginning commitment, here are a few guidelines:

Meditate for Long Enough that You Wish You Could be Anywhere Else

One aspect of our mission is to overcome the tendency to jump ship anytime we feel something unpleasant.

There will always be a part of our mind that seeks pleasure and avoids pain and boredom. This aspect of the mind thinks it's more important to do dishes, pay taxes, or any number of equally boring things but offers relief from the self-imposed torture of meditation.

Getting beyond that discomfort is the jumping-off point for some fundamental brain changes. Don't sell yourself short by doing so little you never have the chance to experience the deeper benefits of concentration practice.

While starting with five minutes is great, especially if you really make those minutes count, stretching it a little longer is recommended. Please recognize that the magic may be right around the corner with just a bit more discomfort and a few more minutes of your time.

Ultimately, 20 minutes is a great beginning goal to stretch to.

What Kind of Timer?

An inexpensive kitchen timer will do the trick.

There are many meditation apps and timers to use with a phone. While those may be useful if you are doing a guided meditation or progressive relaxation, they are not so helpful here.

The phone is a big temptation for most of us these days. The likelihood that you will want to check it is high. Keep it in another room and off if at all possible—no need to be a reactive puppet to every ping and ding coming off that thing.

Of course, if you want a fancy timer that has the whole meditator aesthetic thing going on, that is awesome too, as long as it pretty much does one thing, signals you that the meditation session is over.

Create an Intention

Set the intention and be resolute in your commitment that no matter how it goes, you will continue meditation for the chosen practice time.

Find the Breath

Now that you are seated with a straight spine and have the timer set, begin.

We will use the breath as the primary object of concentration.

There are two things that may complicate finding the breath.

Thing 1. It produces sensations in many parts of the body.

Thing 2. It is tempting to control it or do fancy things with it when you start the practice of finding it.

Where is the Breath?

Option 1. The rim of the nostrils.

Now that you are seated, timed, and prepared, take three deeper and slightly harder breaths to orient you to where the breath is. These will be the only controlled breaths in this practice.

Next, breathe normally. The breath flows in and out freely and with no effort on your part.

Begin to focus your attention on the rims of the nostrils.

Simply notice the feeling of the breath going in and out.

Once an inhalation is through, there will be a pause before the exhalation. Once the exhalation is complete, there will be a pause before the inhalation.

Treat these subtle movements of the breath like targets for your practice.

The mind needs refinement and concentration to notice them.

Be kind and patient as you allow the mind to achieve concentration.

Feel the way the breath moves and touches the skin below the nostrils.

Try not to use any words or mental images.

See if you can simply notice. Putting gentle attention to the subtle sensation of the breath right around the nostrils.

At first, the breaths may be short.

Later, the breaths may be long.

Notice without naming.

Option 2. The rising and falling of the abdomen.

You can also notice the sensation of the breath in the abdomen, as the breath causes the abdomen to rise and fall.

The same principle applies.

Find the breath in the abdomen and observe the breath in the abdomen as it rises and falls.

Notice when it is short and notice when it is long.

Simply Notice.

Abdomen or Nostrils? Where to Focus?

Choose only one for the duration of your meditation practice. After you have tried each a few times, choose your main squeeze to advance in practice with. Being in a committed relationship to a meditation technique allows for depth and precision in practice.

Stick with one or the other for a period of time to see if you are gaining traction in your ability to concentrate. If you have practiced consistently for a week or more and don't seem to be getting it, switch to the other one.

Note.

Focusing on the small space beneath the nostrils lends itself well to refinement and subtlety. It has a sharpening effect on the mind.

Resting attention on the breath in the abdomen is great for when there is emotional turbulence or a distracted mind that has trouble fixating on the more subtle breath underneath the nostrils. This approach can be relaxing. Be careful not to fall asleep!

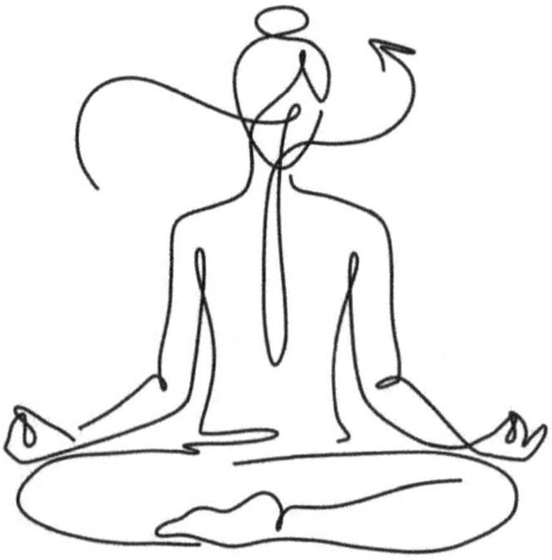

Avoid Manipulation

Whichever you choose, the important point is that you do not direct or manipulate the breath. This is no time to be a control freak. You are a watcher. Nothing more. The breath is doing its thing, and you are spectating.

Put another way, just because it is such an important distinction. *You are not meditating to control the breath. You are meditating to notice it.*

That's it.

Mind Wanders, Bring It Back

Allow your attention to stay focused on the breath, whichever you choose.

You will have some awareness of what's going on in the background. You can stay relaxed and open with that peripheral awareness. We are hardwired to be aware of our surroundings. However, your deliberate attention remains on the breath.

No matter what, until you reach higher states of meditation, your attention will sometimes stray from the meditation object.

Your mind is not faulty for allowing the attention to stray.

Your mind is not bad or dumb or anything like that. Minds will be minds. It's what they do.

With no judgment or frustration, guide your attention back to the breath.

Reinforce the positive. You are able to bring it back. Again and Again.

Keep returning to the breath every time the mind wanders off the meditation object.

Finish

After your timer goes off, you can finish with some sort of grounding, centering, or prayer.

A traditional way to finish meditation is to offer a loving kindness prayer. This is optional but highly recommended.

With deeper experience and growth in meditation, compassion becomes a default setting for how you see the world. By working with your own mind, you will understand that all humans are saddled with the same basic sets of problems. This allows you to feel understanding toward those who may not be the most skillful (that is not to say you need to take their crap, just that you will understand why it is tossed your way).

True compassion is genuine, never forced.

Until compassion bubbles up freely in you, it helps to reinforce this aspect of your nature. This prayer is a good soul balm. This is not a prayer to any deity or outside entity but a general prayer.

In regions of India and Tibet, you will see a similar prayer written on flags that blow in the wind, allowing it to be carried far and wide for everyone.

There are many beautiful versions of this prayer across different traditions, but in a nutshell, it goes like this.

May I be peaceful.

May I be happy.

May I be liberated.

May I share my peace with others.

May all beings be peaceful.

May all beings be happy.

May all beings be liberated.

Feel free to end it with a little bow or hands in prayer position if that feels good to you.

Now you can go about your day!

PART 3.

GOING DEEPER AND UNDERSTANDING THE CONTEXT.

What Comes Next?

The practice taught in part 2 is considered a concentration practice. With that practice, you are working to deliberately bring your attention to a specific point of concentration while moving your mind away from swinging from one thought to another.

From this point forward, our discussion becomes more specific.

Once you have mastered concentration to a decent degree, you will have the ability to direct your meditation practice in various ways, depending on what you prefer to experience. What you emphasize will determine the direction you grow. Think of your practice like a bonsai tree.

Moving forward, the concepts and language will be specifically coming out of the Theravada Buddhist tradition, also referred to as the Insight Tradition. The terms and ideas are from some of the oldest books on meditation, a group of books called the Pali canon. Pali was the ancient language spoken by Gautama the Buddha, the person we now commonly refer to as the Buddha.

As mentioned earlier in this book, in Buddhism, there are religious aspects among followers experienced as rites and rituals. There are also practical aspects of meditation training that have come from those same traditions that modern popular culture folds into itself as the phrases and concepts we think about when we consider meditation and mindfulness. It is possible and even encouraged to practice meditation and have a deeper, more nuanced practice without ever worshiping in a religious way.

The texts and practices from the origin of Buddhism shared throughout the centuries are still very informative in the practical sense because they show us not only what is possible in meditation but also how to direct our attention in the most skillful ways.

At First Nothing Needs to Change

Believe it or not, you could keep doing the practice presented in part 2, using those same instructions during every session, for hours and hours, for the rest of your life.

If you were to take that approach without adding any other practice, something would eventually shift in your meditation, and you would start to enter into meditative states called Jhanas.

In full transparency, though the practice of concentration is simple, a set of instructions repeated again and again, only working with it for a few minutes a day, is unlikely to yield an experience of the states I am about to discuss.

If you are not ready to commit 20–30 minutes of dedicated meditation time a day or more, that is fine. This may be something that you come back to read when you are ready. If you read now, you may find that this inspires you to increase your practice time.

What's a Jhana?

Jhana is a Pali term that translates to mean "meditation." Jhana is usually understood to mean a meditative state in which the meditator is profoundly still and in perfect concentration. Multiple Jhana's have been identified and have different qualities as you advance in practice.

Advanced meditators from many different traditions have mapped out these states. No matter the specific differences in any given tradition, the results of concentration practice tend to follow a somewhat predictable trajectory. These stages that people advance through are called Jhanas.

Like rungs on a ladder, these states are progressive. In the tradition we are talking about here, there are eight concentration Jhanas, the first three of which you may encounter with a home practice.

If you start feeling something new and unusual in your state of awareness within the context of meditation, this is likely a Jhana.

The Jhana Ladder

One way to think about progress in meditation states is that as you grow and access these higher states of consciousness, you simultaneously let go of aspects of normal waking consciousness.

Access concentration could be considered the phase in which you become able to even find the ladder. You need to be able to tame the mind wandering enough to have moments of freedom when you are not engaged with the content of your thoughts at all. If you have them, you don't follow them. You are able to return to that breath with increased ease.

Once you get into the Jhanas and onto the ladder, you will sense that your concentration has shifted. In general, there is a feeling of quiet and peace as you move away from noisy thinking.

As you move up the ladder, you drop some baggage, and as you get higher, you start picking up new skillful modes of operation. First, you let go, then you add, and then with each addition of a new way of operating, you let go more deeply.

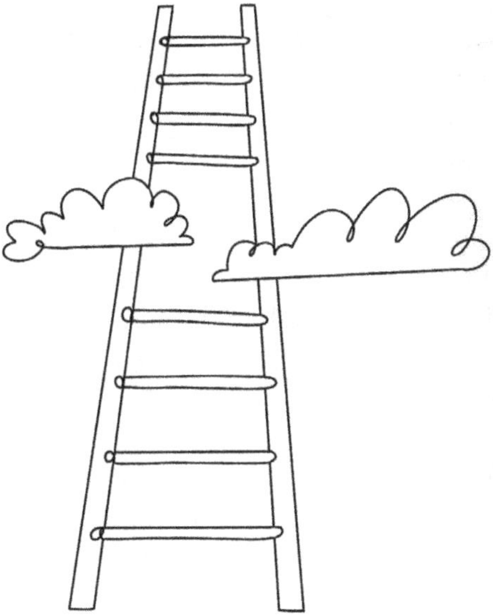

The Concentration Jhanas 1-4

As you progress in your ability to refine your concentration, the meditative states become increasingly subtle. You will notice in the following description that the first three Jhanas are identified by qualities that are let go of as you pass through the stages. After the third Jhana, new qualities are added.

The first Jhana is characterized by the five following qualities, translated from Pali.

- **VITAKKA.** The normal process of discursive thinking in which the mind passes from one subject to another. This is what we think of as "monkey mind," the way our minds work before we learn how to control the incessant flow of thinking.

- **VICĀRA.** The sustained application of the mind on the object of meditation. This is where we finally are able to settle the mind in concentration, even if only for a few fleeting moments.

- **PITI.** The mental factor that perceives the quality of the object but is still non-neutral and able to color the mind with opinion. This is where we can notice something for what it is, breath as breath, for example, but we are not completely neutral yet.

- **SUKHA.** Happiness, pleasure, ease, joy, or bliss. This quality is the expansive and joyful aspect of a Jhana state and can result in a whole body feeling of ease.

- **EKAGGATA.** Tranquility of mind. A calm and present state of equanimity.

The second Jhana drops the Vitakka and Vicara, as the meditator moves into a state that includes only the following;

- **PITI**
- **SUKHA**
- **EKAGGATA**

The third Jhana drops the Piti and maintains the last two aspects;

- **SUKHA**
- **EKAGGATA**

The fourth Jhana keeps only Ekagatta from that previous list and adds a new aspect.

- **EKAGATTA**
- **UPEKKHA.** Stability in the face of the fluctuations of worldly fortune. This is a state of unshakeable inner poise not influenced by gain or loss, honor or dishonor, praise or blame, pleasure or pain.

The Concentration Jhanas 5-8

5. Base of Boundless Space
6. Base of Boundless Consciousness
7. Base of Nothingness
8. Base of Neither Perception nor Non-Perception

I've listed the higher concentration Jhanas here, but please note that getting into serious practice is best accomplished in a supportive environment with an experienced teacher. To be successful at navigating these states without getting lost in the ever enticing ego trip means that you need perspective and grounding in the reality that what looks like enlightenment to you may look like a kindergarten stage for someone with more experience.

These higher states can make you feel high, for lack of a better word. The highness of them is even implied in the names! Coming back down to earth to carry on with life is important and can be difficult for those who choose to spend much time in these states.

Exploration of the 5-8 Jhanas is typically taken on by meditation practitioners who want to stay on the path of concentration practice and who will be working with various objects of meditation such as mantras (words or repeated sayings) or Kasina practices (where concentration is focused on an outer object such as a candle flame or color). There are entire traditions devoted to exploring concentration Jhanas, should you want to work specifically this way.

A Fork in the Road

This is a turning point in your decision-making about which kind of practice you want to pursue. I have taken the path of Insight by choosing to stick with Vipassana meditation. However, you may resonate with other practices such as Kasina, Mantra, or Yogic Drishti. These will keep you on the path of growth in what is still considered concentration.

No matter what direction you take, the skills you have developed will serve you well.

Insight Practice can be started as soon as the first Jhana but takes a more defined departure around the fourth Jhana. By choosing Insight as our primary practice, we commit to changing how we meditate. Brain studies found that the mental states of Vipassana meditators (the meditation approach emphasized in the Insight tradition) were more likely

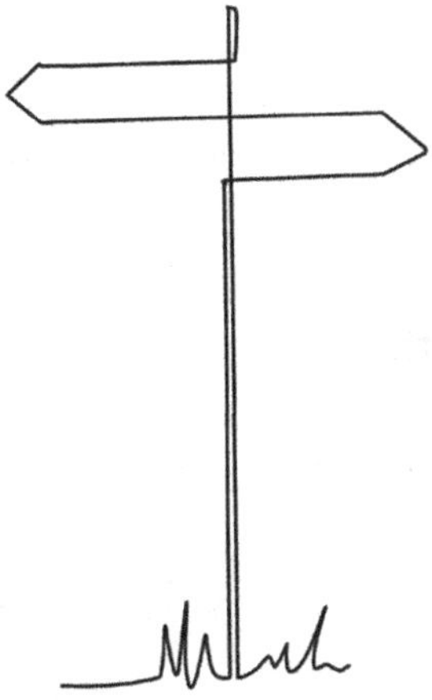

to increase Gamma waves. My humble opinion is that the departure from concentration practices after the third Jhana differentiates the Vipassana practice emphasized in the insight traditions from other meditation traditions and leads to the increase in Gamma waves.

Later, we will get into more specifics about what Vipassana practice is. For now, back to those first three Jhana's, the ones most likely to pertain to your home practice.

What's it like to Experience a Jhana?

As a beginning meditator, your thoughts may seem too wild to tame. Eventually, with repeated practice, you overcome this difficulty. At this point, you are able to steady the mind completely on your breath. As though the attention is fused to it, not entirely separate from it.

This is around when you pass through the state of access concentration, where you have enough ability for your mind to shift. Using that stabilized attention that you cultivated with practice, you allow your mind to experience a change in the way that attention feels.

It goes a little like this. There you are, doing your daily practice as always. Bring attention to the breath. Mind wanders. Bring attention back to the breath. Mind wanders.

And then poof. You are suddenly totally focused and in flow with no mind wandering for a period of time.

This new way of experiencing your attention is likely the first Jhana. Unless you intend to focus on how to cultivate the Jhanas deliberately, chances are you will be phasing in and out of the first three Jhanas regularly. One of the features of these states is that they are not permanent and stable. So, the first feels a little wobbly, like you could easily return to that busy mind, the second, less so, and the third feels the most stable, with a higher degree of peace and steadiness.

It's Probably One of the First Three Jhanas if You Feel Good

Once you get past the phase where you feel like you are always wrangling and fighting against your thoughts, you find yourself in a lovely flow state that feels a little buzzy and nice. Your body and mind will feel at ease, and you may start to see a sort of light show behind your eyes. You feel like you could sit there all day, but it still has a quality of ending easily. Ultimately, the fact that it is so tenuous will create some frustration. As you progress through the Jhanas, the sense of stability in that state increases.

All Jhana's may have a similar feeling as other flow states we achieve in life when we are completely absorbed in an activity or pursuit. Playing a sport, instrument, or artistic pursuit have a similar quality. It is important to note some differences between Jhana and ordinary flow states.

The first is that a Jhana is wholesome. The second is that it is within the context of meditation.

It is possible to have a sense of concentration while engaged in things that are not wholesome—for example, greed, lust, desire, and the thrill of the chase. Being obsessed with something we want and going after it with a single-minded focus is concentrated but will not yield a Jhana experience.

Even wholesome activities such as cooking, gardening, or painting that allow for complete focus and flow are still not Jhana states. Jhanas are wholesome flow states that happen in the context of meditation.

If this shift in the way your mind and body feels is created by directed, sustained, and wholesome attention within the context of meditation, it is a Jhana.

Jhanas Feel like a Reward for all of Your Hard Work on the Cushion

Early Jhanas, the first three rungs on that ladder, tend to have a quality of joy, bodily pleasure, and peacefulness. They feel good.

Life can be hard. Having the ability to take a mental break and hang out in Jhana states is one of the ways that meditation reduces stress, and benefits overall health. You can keep growing in your ability to enjoy these states, returning again and again.

Practice Without Imitation

Before discussing Jhanas, please note that this is not a fake until you make it sort of scenario. Getting into any meditative state higher than access concentration happens because your practice has facilitated the opportunity for it to happen.

Through repeated practice, you make these chance encounters possible. They are not available through force.

The opportunity to experience the state of silence and stillness in perception doesn't happen because you set out to make it happen. It isn't because you hear about it from a friend and are imitating what you heard. These states bubble up naturally as a result of consistent and diligent practice.

The Maps Help You Know the Terrain

Meditators in various traditions throughout time have documented these stages. From Vipassana to Mayahana to Yogic traditions, those that have come before us have left records of what is to be expected on the meditative journey. These experiences, described in both books and lectures, have become maps that help meditators understand the terrain of changes that occur with sincere practice.

These maps can tempt us to shift our focus away from what our own practice is. It is common to forget to come back to this moment in meditation once we know something else is possible. It's enticing to skip the boring part that feels like work and just jump into the bliss pool and stay there.

Even though you know something is possible in meditation, it does you absolutely zero good to push yourself in a way that you think will produce an experience. This can set you up to unintentionally manufacture the experience, missing out on what unfolds for you. Jhanas are not unique in that they have been documented as predictable states that you pass through as a meditator, but they are unique in that your exact experience will be unique to you.

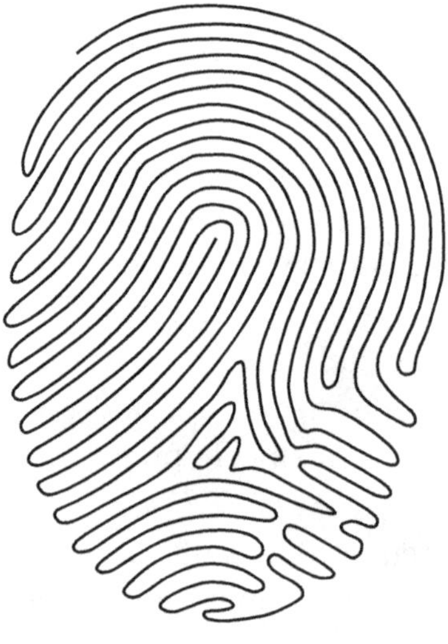

It's Not a Competition, Not Even with Yourself

Creating a competitive or forced attitude in meditation is a risk that comes from having some knowledge of advanced stages.

There's a subtle difference between an experience happening because it really happened and an experience happening because you knew it might happen.

This is your own gig. Your growth rate is dependent on many factors, none the same as anyone else's.

Another truth is that goals in practice can be a slippery slope, especially for certain types of people that enjoy competition and have perfectionist tendencies. I would think of the maps and terrain of meditation practice as similar to getting ready to take a trip to somewhere you have never been. Some may prefer to map out a very specific itinerary from home. Once they arrive at the new place, they realize that the museum they planned to visit is now closed, or the weather is completely ruining the plans for a certain hike. The actual experience in front of the person has priority over what was listed on the itinerary. It absolutely is more important than replicating the experience their friend or other travel resource shared.

It's like that with meditation practice as well. Jhana's and higher states are like notes from someone else's travel journal.

Talking About Jhanas may be Frowned Upon

Many teachers, especially in monasteries in Southeast Asia, will be tight-lipped or vague about what to expect in meditation. But having some knowledge of where you are going without forcing yourself to get there has value too. In modern pop culture, this notion of practicing without goals may have been taken too far in that people don't seem to have any sense of direction and may not have any context for understanding the potential of meditation as it is, but quickly get caught up mistaking it as another form of psychological healing like therapy.

These are actual conversations from a silent meditation retreat in India (my first). I was learning a whole system of meditation very practically with no sense of direction. I now see how important that was for the reasons I mentioned above. The training emphasized that meditation is something that you must do for yourself. No one else can do it for you.

In keeping with that advice, my teacher would smartly only focus on the nuts and bolts of the practice when I was able to speak with him (he was one of two people I was allowed to speak to).

No matter what I said in an interview, his answer was always a question. "Can you find the breath?"

Me: "I saw some lights and felt a buzzing bliss." (probably Jhana state)

Teacher: "Can you find the breath."

Me: "I was feeling a lot of grief and couldn't sit still." (struggling with psychological content in between Jhana state)

Teacher: "Can you find the breath?"

Me: "On break, I was surrounded by a group of monkeys who took mercy on me when the alpha monkey chased them away. Should I do something about the monkeys?" (dealing with life in India)

Teacher: "Speak with the female manager. Can you find the breath?"

That was it.

The only thing that matters is proper practice.

The Reason to Mention Jhanas

So, you may wonder why even learn about Jhanas if it's best not to force yourself into them or think about them.

The reason here is that should you start experiencing Jhana states, it will change the way you concentrate, and it may be harder for you to orient to the subtle sensation below the nostrils, but not for the same reason it happened before.

Before you achieved access concentration, you would be in a

state of mind where it was difficult to quiet the mind enough to pinpoint the breath as an object of meditation.

This time, you may struggle to orient to the breath because you are suddenly in a zone of quiet and bliss where the attention feels more diffuse. The mind noise has died down, and you are still concentrating, but without the same need for deliberate directed-ness. It may surprise you that you find no need to redirect the mind as you had previously.

You may want to return to the practice you were doing before but find it difficult. Putting attention on the breath will feel futile. It's ok at this point to just stay in that state. A wholesome state of pleasant flow that does not feel rigid or forced.

Though the results are repeatable at this stage, they are not guaranteed to happen every time you sit.

Like All Things In Life, These States are Not Permanent

Once your meditation session ends, you likely will have a nice calm feeling. Clear-minded brightness will permeate at least part of your day, that is, until you step in dog pee, trip on a lego, or run into a gossipy neighbor.

Until you reach the final stages on the path, the world will inevitably ***harsh your mellow.***

This is the very reason to consider moving on to another approach. Vipassana. The goal of Vipassana meditation is to take that concentration and apply it differently, with the intent of making permanent changes in how your mind behaves.

Concentration Practice in Context

What we just learned and practiced is training in concentration. This could be it. Plenty of meditation traditions only operate in the realm of concentration. The terrain of Concentration Jhanas alone could take a lifetime to master. However, once we establish concentration, there is another option.

After you have mastered concentration, experienced early Jhanic states, and have ridden the waves of meditative bliss only to come out and step in dog piss, you may start to wonder. So what? Why do I bother? Even though I'm certainly calmer than the next guy, life still gets me down, and I am not the oh-so-special superhero I thought meditation would turn me into.

In the tradition of Insight Meditation, concentration is one of three parts.

Once we establish the ability to still the mind to notice subtlety, we can shift the practice in another direction—vipassana practice. Vipassana's belief system is the path to ultimate liberation (enlightenment) from the reactive ups and downs of normal consciousness. From the perspective of this tradition, concentration is important so that you can start and maintain the practice of Vipassana. Still, it is not an end itself since you won't be able to sustain Jhanas off the cushion.

A Three Part Training

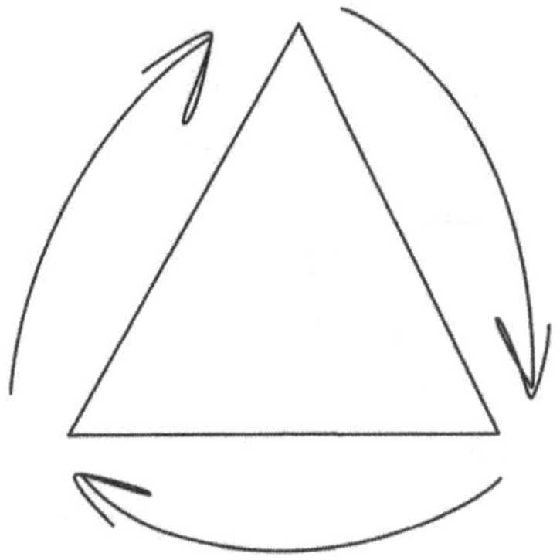

Insight meditation emphasizes three types of training.

1. Sila. Morality
2. Samadhi. Concentration
3. Panna. Wisdom

These three parts are interdependent, all equally essential to achieving mastery. The goal of meditation from this perspective is ultimate liberation, which means freedom from the cycle of suffering caused by attachment to the notion of a fixed and permanent self.

I know. Deep.

Morality and concentration are the two aspects of the three that beginners can practice.

The wisdom aspect of training involves a different approach to meditation, Vipassana, an endeavor that usually isn't taken on until you can concentrate on the refined and subtle aspects of the breath.

Concentration practice and morality practice focus on reducing suffering, whereas Vipassana practice focuses on the ultimate mental liberation.

There are levels to this thing.

Morality: One of the Three Parts of Insight Practice: Life Off the Cushion

Morality has a specific set of codes of conduct in formal insight meditation training. One set is for monks, and one set is for householders.

The five precepts for householders (those of us not living in monastic settings) are as follows:

1. Abstain from taking life.
2. Abstain from taking that which is not given.

3. Abstain from sensuous misconduct.
4. Abstain from false speech.
5. Abstain from intoxicants as they tend to cloud the mind.

What these meant in the context of ancient life in India, Tibet, or Burma differed from what they mean for us today.

For example, one of the early documents outlined that a person could engage in sensuous misconduct by having sexual intercourse with a concubine who once carried a load on her head or someone acquired through a ceremony that involved dipping hands in water.

These are unlikely to concern you when you consider a sexual partner.

Equality and consent are probably more pressing issues in modern times.

We need different metrics for what constitutes good conduct.

Building Morality: Starting with Where You Are

Not only will meditation help you live a happier life, but also living a wholesome life will strengthen meditation.

The word morality can bring up unsavory connotations for

some. We are at a point in history where trauma and persecution in the name of religion are genuine issues. There are plenty of us who may have felt rejected or judged by the "moral police" in our families and communities, or who have felt shame based not on some terrible thing that we did but rather that shame was the habit adopted by our family of origin.

Dividing our notions of morality from religious upbringing and dogma can be challenging.

In the context of growth in meditation, think of it as more of a practical issue beyond choosing to be a decent human for obvious reasons, such as the ability to participate in society without being a menace, having stability in work and relationships, and basically living a happy drama free life. Wholesomeness will make your meditation practice much stronger.

Meditation does lead to a clear mind, which helps tremendously in making less emotionally erratic decisions in life. That said, getting deep into meditative states is much harder if you have been engaging in activities that lead to emotional or mental chaos. To begin meditating, you do not need to be "perfect" in any sense of the world. However, with sincere practice, you will very likely start to find out where you could apply skillful boundaries in how you engage with the world.

Self Reflection Is a Gift to Your Future.

The life we have now is the result of chain reactions that began in the past—recent or long ago. To make a break in this chain reaction of events, we need to stop generating new problems for ourselves. Even as we are still living out the consequences of the past, we can take a stand for a peaceful future by suspending our reactive tendencies.

Morality in the context of meditation practice is a very specific and personal issue. As you investigate reality more deeply, the vibrational results of your actions become more evident.

The karmic chain of reaping and sowing becomes evident with specific and felt immediacy. This is not because someone else has told you what is right and wrong, but because it is so clear when your own thoughts, words, or actions, have contributed to your own ongoing misery. When you show up to the cushion every day, you get immediate feedback on how well you are doing in life. Are you hungover? Are you regretting an intimate encounter? Are you replaying an unfortunate conversation that stirred you up?

Without shame or regret, you check yourself before you wreck yourself.

Morality While on Retreat Vs. Morality at Home

In monasteries and serious meditation retreat centers, there are strict rules of conduct that support intense meditation practice. The vows of silence keep you from lying or gossiping, the vows of abstinence from intoxicants are supported by the lack of available intoxicants, and the vows around sexual misconduct are easy to uphold when there is no contact between participants.

In daily life, this can be much murkier.

Depending on how seriously you want to take a meditation practice, it can take a while to make the commitment needed to go deeper in practice.

What feels wholesome to you? At this point in history, most of us are too sophisticated to have someone tell us what to do. We can understand that actions create consequences. With a mind made more evident through practice, you will likely be primed to see when an unskilled decision is in front of you. Getting older and more experienced helps too!

Since meditation is about "waking up," it serves to create a life that you want to wake up in.

Instead of "bringing sexy back," let's bring wholesome back.

Not dogmatic wholesomeness—just wholesomeness that recognizes the impact of your actions and habits of mind.

What kind of ripple effect are you having on the world around you, and can you shift that without shaming or judging yourself for not getting it perfect every time?

Wisdom: Vipassana Approach to Meditation

This leg of the journey is about understanding reality at a fundamental level. Typically, our minds keep us from experiencing reality's oscillating and ever-changing nature to preserve our sense of identity and importance. It's a sort of jacked-up overprotective survival mechanism that ensures we keep reproducing and creating empires.

The fundamental truth of reality is that nothing in the field of your experience is lasting, personal, or ultimately satisfying. This is where we get into non-attachment.

It is understandably uncomfortable to overthink our impermanence. Yet there it is, always lurking as a truth we "know" but mostly ignore.

The technique of Vipassana meditation seeks to create a practice where the meditator understands these truths through direct experience, allowing for the meditator to cross over into a state of mind that allows for permanent liberation from the ups and downs caused by attachment to a separate sense of self as a permanent and fixed entity.

Vipassana Practice Makes use of the Concentration that was Cultivated

In the Insight tradition I trained in, the Vipassana technique was introduced after approximately 40 hours of concentration practice since the practice of Vipassana requires the ability to direct the refined concentration that we cultivated in part 2.

It was discouraged that people try learning Vipassana outside the context of retreat, possibly because it can be very intense as it tends to potentially expose the main chasm between what is typically perceived and what is happening under the surface of all of our protective mechanisms.

A General Description of Vipassana

Vipassana takes the concentration you have established and directs it at other areas of the body. There are various ways to apply the shift in concentration, from full-body scanning to highlighting a certain body part with your attention. Still, the point is that you direct that particular and refined attention to an aspect of the body and then remain calm and attentive as you watch it do what it does.

No matter how uncomfortable, painful, pleasant, or lovely, you treat all sensations equally as they arise and pass away.

An example from my practice is this: once introduced to

Vipassana meditation, is common practice to have sitting sessions where the meditator resolves to sit perfectly still without shifting the body. In this case, it was for an hour. (Please note. I am not recommending you do this in-home practice unless you have been trained or are in a supportive atmosphere).

As I sat for an hour, my knee started burning. I had a strong resolve to sit with it. I also had strongly established concentration at this point. I practiced properly, observing the sensation without labels or judgment. In this particular instance, I was able to remain non-reactive. The sensation in my knee swirled and changed. It grew hot, then cold. It oscillated. I observed the knee as a shifting group of subatomic particles, diffuse and unrelated to me. Not mine, not my pain, not my knee, nothing at all except for an impersonal shifting experience. I observed that everything about that experience was still changing without me changing anything. (also, by the way, the pain disappeared without me moving my legs).

The Resilience to be with Life as It Is

With Vipassana practice, you run straight into facing life as it is, not as you want it to be.

This is advanced level truthfulness and quite a departure from our usual way of approaching problems. Rather than fix or change what is unpleasant or chase what is pleasant, we learn to watch without reaction or judgment. With this practice, we accomplish this understanding at an advanced cellular level.

Once concentration has been established and getting into Jhana states are the norm, it's probably time to sacrifice your luxury vacation for a meditation retreat. You'll find some resources at the end of this book. I don't endorse working with Vipassana on your own until you have had training from a living teacher or community. This is the main reason I am not teaching it here. Also, it's outside the scope of my job description!

Where Does Mindfulness Fit In?

I will admit that it was embarrassing for me when clients started talking about their "mindfulness" practices, and I didn't get what they were talking about. I thought, as a long-term meditator, I must be missing something. What practice were they actually doing? As it turns out, it was just as vague for everyone I asked as it was for me.

Mindfulness is derived from the ancient Pali word Sati and became popular in Western culture as part of modern meditation training to help treat psychological stress.

What makes it vague is that it has become understood and named as a system in and of itself. When considered as part of Insight Meditation, it helps us see it as a technique applied to our other practices.

Mindfulness is Applied when Developing Concentration

Strictly speaking, mindfulness goes hand in hand with concentration practice. Like two wings on one bird, mindfulness and concentration in balance lead to the specific type of meditative awareness we achieve when the mind is perfectly still but without the rigidity of forced concentration.

Mindfulness is the aspect of our awareness that keeps us on track in meditation. The exact moment that we realize the mind has wandered, and we get back to the business of bringing conscious awareness to the breath.

Mindfulness is pre-verbal and precognitive awareness. You can only catch true mindfulness in a split second before the mind has taken on the task of naming and categorizing an experience.

Mindfulness is the moment exactly before you add any extras. We use mindfulness to catch ourselves and to remain present.

Mindfulness Off the Cushion is Practiced when Refining Morality

Mindfulness is the moment before our experience becomes solid in our minds before we give something a name or a predesignated assignment of good or bad. That tiny moment offers us a departure from being swept up in the typical thought patterns of our minds. It's one moment when we are interacting with life directly and without interpretation.

In life, we can make an effort to exercise mindfulness as an aspect of training in morality. By being aware of what we are doing and our surroundings, by continuously bringing our conscious minds out of fantasy and into the exact moment of our reality as we shop, cook, clean, spend time with loved ones, work, and move around, allows for a natural wholesomeness and is likely to foster decisions that lead us where we want to go.

Mindfulness is also Practiced when the Mind Wanders During Vipassana

Having built up the ability to refine the attention through concentration practice that also relies on mindfulness, you move into Vipassana which can be seen as mindfulness and concentration used in a very specific way.

Mindfulness is still present when practicing Vipassana, but that awareness can get more detailed and specific, still exercising the sharpness of mind that catches itself before you start running away from unpleasantness or chasing toward pleasantness. You see yourself before you forget to investigate sensations from a neutral stance.

Insight Practice Includes Training in Morality, Concentration, and Wisdom

In summary, it's essential to understand how intertwined these aspects of practice are, no matter how advanced you get. Even though concentration, once well established, will be relatively easy to get into, there are times when it will fluctuate, and you may need to focus back on stabilizing concentration. Also, there will be times when life is tumultuous, and you may need to focus on bringing peace back to your daily life, focusing on morality. All of these aspects of training fit together and strengthen one another.

Returning to the Simple

It may feel like we have come a long way from my early assertion that meditation is simple.

But really, it is.

Think about how little you need to know to start practicing! Just those instructions in part 2.

The essential equipment for the practice is always with you. A body. A mind. An object of concentration that is part of your body.

You don't need to do any more than that to gain some mastery over your mental chatter.

However, I hope this book has inspired you to understand the context of that practice and to have fun with its potential to help you create more peace in your mind and your life, should you commit more time and training.

By keeping the scope of your practice limited to the stage you are in while also being aware that more is possible, you will be inspired to sit down and make a sincere effort without being burdened by the frustration that you can't do it or are doing it wrong.

Concentration may be the first step in insight practice, and it also may be the only step you need to take to feel fulfilled in your practice.

In summary, I would like you to know that you can start a serious meditation practice at home. Serious in the sense that you apply a specific way of meditating repeatedly and consistently enough to grow beyond the"my mind is too busy!" phase.

You can achieve a calm and quiet mind, even if only for a few minutes a day. Those few minutes will also inspire you to increase the peace in all of the other moments. Your peace will inspire those around you.

Should you feel intrigued by the glimpse of what the Jhanas offer and ultimately be interested in learning Vipassana, I wish you the very best in devoting more time and training to your practice.

You can always learn more about meditation and choose to

go further with your practice. By taking responsibility for your mind, you are already going against the grain of the majority.

All you need to do is start. You just need some time each day, a body and a mind. You have everything you need. It is already with you.

Now, I encourage you to put down this book and find a seat on your cushion!

Resources

This book was written from my limited vantage point, based on teachers I have worked with, books I have read, and my interpretation of all of those influences as I take a seat on my meditation cushion.

If anything here goes against what you were taught, is confusing, or doesn't make sense, or even if everything makes total sense, I encourage you to dig deeper and learn more as you go about your practice.

Here are some books that may help you.

Mindfulness In Plain English. Bhante Henepola Gunaratana

The Mind Illuminated. Culadasa (John Yates, PhD), Mathew Immergut PhD, Jeremy Graves.

Practical Insight Meditation. Mahasi Sayadaw

Mastering The Core Teaching of the Buddha. Daniel M. Ingram

Courses

At a certain point, you may want advanced training, and the opportunity to practice with more support.

Here are some reputable places to do that.

Vipassana Meditation as taught by S.N. Goenka (worldwide)
www.dhamma.org

Insight Meditation Society (Massachusetts, U.S.A.)
www.dharma.org

Buddhist Insight Network
www.buddhistinsightnetwork.org

Acknowledgments

Thank you Justin and Laila, not only for putting up with me, but also for encouraging me as I figured out how to write a book. Your contribution and support in keeping our household peaceful mean the world to me. Beasley, I know you tried your best.

Lindsey, Alex, Woz, and the team at Get It Done, I would not have been able to do this without your guidance. It has been a blast working with you. The process of bringing this book from vague idea, to something with a cover and pages, amazes me. Your team first made the impossible seem possible, and then made it seem easy, even when it wasn't.

Ru, Tarah, Stephanie, and many other clients and friends, I loved speaking with you about your meditation experiences. I hope that this book helps you find the right practice for you.

Vig, Lucia, Lamay, thank you for being living examples of what serious meditation practice looks like.

Mom, Ryan, Jack, and Linda, Thank you for being the type of family that has unwavering faith in me.

Sade, Darius, Jocylyn, Kim and Leticia, thank you for welcoming me into your family.

Demitra, Katie, Laura, Maria, Monique, Radha, Heidi, Lisa, and the squad ladies. Friends. I can't believe I'm lucky to have so many good ones. Thank you for saying you will read this book even if you have zero interest in meditation. .

All my acupuncture clients, going back to the beginning of my time in practice. Thank you for being open to Chinese medicine, and for putting your trust in me. By working with you, I have been able to see how all people share the same basic struggles, dealing with the limitations of a body and mind, and how we can still be happy and healthy even with those limitations.

CPSIA information can be obtained
at www.ICGtesting.com
Printed in the USA
BVHW041050171022
649607BV00002B/25

9 781956 989120